Intermittent Fasting

The Safe Guide to Long Lasting Weight Loss

Miranda Jaso

Table of Contents

liable for any hardship or damages that may befall them after undertaking information described herein.

Additionally, the information in the following pages is intended only for informational purposes and should thus be thought of as universal. As befitting its nature, it is presented without assurance regarding its prolonged validity or interim quality. Trademarks that are mentioned are done without written consent and can in no way be considered an endorsement from the trademark holder.

Introduction

Congratulations on downloading *Intermittent Fasting: The safe guide to long-lasting weight loss* and thank you for doing so.

The following chapters will discuss different types of fasting and why intermittent fasting is a good choice for losing weight and keeping it off. The chapters will also cover how the body responds to fasting and the science behind the results. The information here is presented in a manner to decipher the scientific research for the every-day person. It attempts to guide you through the proven benefits of intermittent fasting, how to fast and even provide a comprehensive Q&A to answer some of the most common questions you may wonder about.

When you are deciding to make a major life change, it is important to do so with full knowledge of how it will work and what it is founded upon. The great news is that there is a long history of intermittent and regular fasting. The bad news? There are limited scientific trials with human participants. This means the application of this amazing lifestyle can be interpreted and adapted in various ways because there is no "proven" method that works for everyone. In reality, this probably will never happen as each individual is different and will require a tailored approach. This is why Chapter 7 is dedicated to explaining some of the more common methods of intermittent fasting, providing tips and proposed schedules to help you be successful at it.

You may encounter several nay-sayers when you discuss this form of weight loss and management strategy. To help you guard against their "advice," refer to Chapter 8, where you will be able to dispel almost any myth out there on intermittent fasting.

There are plenty of books on this subject on the market, thanks again for choosing this one! Every effort was made to ensure it is full of as much useful information as possible, please enjoy!

Chapter 1:
History of Fasting

When a person does not eat or drink or abstains from both for a variety of reasons, including ethical, ritualistic, religious, or health reasons, they are fasting. The length of abstaining can vary from years to just a few hours, and it can include full fasting or partial fasting. It can even be intermittent, such as one day on and one day off. This dietary lifestyle has been used since antiquity and has been promoted by physicians, religions, and cultures. Cultures can be large like a country or it can be smaller communities within, such as groups with initiation practices involving fasting or hunters. It has been a form of protest by several groups who are bringing awareness to political, social, or ethical causes that they feel have been violated.

There can be some confusion regarding the difference between "starving yourself" and fasting. It is important to keep in mind that starving is not deliberate. It cannot be controlled. Fasting is a choice. Never intertwine these two terms. Fasting is actually something that occurs every day. Consider the word "Breakfast." The key parts of this word are "break" and "fast." You are fasting while you sleep and are now breaking that by eating food in the morning.

When trying to lose weight, the diet and lifestyle options out there can seem endless. But to truly lose weight and keep it off, the solution is not found in the latest-and-greatest trend; it is in the tried-and-true. This means avoiding the "miracle" pills and "cures" that are promoted and look to the past to find the solutions that have worked for hundreds of centuries. One of the most basic health and wellness traditions in history is fasting. Almost every culture and religion has practiced this form of lifestyle.

History of Fasting

The founder of medicine, Hippocrates, developed many treatment plans that have founded the way we treat patients today. Some of his treatment plans included fasting. He believed that eating during an illness only fed the disease. Plutarch, an ancient historian, and writer, also believed that fasting should be used to heal people. Aristotle, Plato's student, believed in fasting, just as his teacher did. The basis of this belief stemmed from the observation of animal behavior. When animals become sick they naturally want to abstain from eating. This is also true in humans. Our human nature when ill is to stop eating. It becomes repulsive to use, sometimes. With this concept, it can be concluded that fasting is as deep-rooted as humankind itself. More modern supporters of fasting for medical purposes include one of the founders of Western medicine and toxicology's founder, Philip Paracelsus. Even Benjamin Franklin described fasting as one of the best medicines. Consider the old wife's tale, "Feed a cold, starve a fever." This concept has been in practice for health for a long time and continues to this day.

Another reason for fasting is to improve the brain's function. The Greeks discovered that eating large quantities of food made the mind sluggish. We now understand that this is because blood is being diverted to digestion functions from the brain, leaving it less alert and creating an overall feeling in your body of fatigue. In the 19th century, this idea of using fasting as "therapy" to improve the mind became popular. Dr. Hebert Shelton was one of the most well-known physicians to prescribe and monitor the fasting movement of thousands of people to treat a host of illnesses, including mental improvement. The 1920's were a booming era for many things across the globe, including fasting as therapy. While modern Western medicine has pushed this concept aside in current American culture, it is still practiced frequently in other parts of the world, like Germany and the United Kingdom.

Religions have used fasting as a method of cleansing or purifying the soul or body. Almost every major religion includes fasting as part of their religious practice. The healing property of fasting was shared among religious leaders like Muhammed, Jesus Christ, and Buddha. They believed in the deep spiritual benefit to the body. Fasting in the Buddhist culture is commonly practiced with a single, morning meal and nothing until the following day. Greek Orthodox Christians will choose to fast throughout the year, consuming only water for days or weeks. They can fast for up to 200 days through the year. During Ramadan, Muslims fast from the time the sun rises to when it sets again. This practice is one of the most scientifically researched fasting traditions. Muhammed encouraged fasting on specific days of the week, specifically Monday and Thursday. Yom Kippur, the Day of Atonement in Judaism, includes several fasting days. Roman Catholics and Eastern Orthodox choose a form of fasting during Lent.

Choosing to fast for weight loss has been included in all various forms of fasting's history, from medical purposes to mental. Obesity is considered a medical condition that requires a doctor's supervision, and the prescription of fasting as a way to control weight has been used for many years. Other concepts include weight gain as a symptom of mental thoughts processes. Things such as "emotional eater" or "bored eating" are considered learned behaviors that can be rectified by using fasting to "retrain" the mind.

It is evident that this lifestyle has withstood the test of centuries worth of medical and religious advances and been supported by some of the most influential people of the ages.

History of Intermittent Fasting

The concept of Intermittent Fasting, or IF, refers to the fasting diets and the time frame between fasting periods. There are various versions of this type of fasting that have been used for centuries. This form of fasting is possibly one of the most well-utilized forms of fasting and can be traced back to the time of hunting and gathering. For example, when they harvested or hunted for food, they would restrict their eating between days to make the food last longer. This self-control also ensured the ancient humans were able to remain lean and strong. The fat oxidation is the premise of why today this form is used to lower weight and lose unwanted fat.

Later, physicians and religious leaders encouraged IF to improve health and spiritual well-being. For example, Lent is a fast restricted to 40 days once per year. Ramadan is an IF that requires food restriction during daylight hours for a period of time. Doctors will ask patients to fast for several hours before tests or surgeries.

Now, there is a rise in popularity again for intermittent fasting. Examples of popular modern IF's include the 5/2 diet, where a person eats normally for 5 days and fasts for 2 days, or modified foods for a period of time, like an all juice diet.

Chapter 2:
Body changes During Fasting

As our bodies enter the fasting state, about 5 hours after eating, hormone fluctuations are spurred by dropping insulin levels. The body begins generating energy from the fat stores once the glucose is burned up. This change to fat burning from glucose is the primary benefit of fasting for weight loss. The time it takes for a body to make this switch can vary but in general, it takes about 12 hours. Some of the variables include:

1. If your body is used to switching to a fat burning mode.

2. The amount of glucose needed to be burned. This can be contingent on your muscle and liver's ability to hold on to glycogen and the number of carbohydrates consumed.

3. Your activity levels during the period of fasting, which determines the speed with which your body uses up the stores of glycogen.

When your body begins to dip into the fats stores and your body begins to burn fat, your body begins to show changes. These changes can be dramatic. The internal change of a decreased insulin level is the result of the fall in glucose levels in the blood. This makes the body's cells turn into a repair phase from a growth phase. The liver controls the risk of the glucose levels dropping too low because it kicks up its production of glucose. The cells become sensitive to the drop in insulin making it hardened to resistance to insulin and improved insulin tolerance.

The reason glucose is critical to weight loss is that when there is an increase in the secretion of glucagon burning of fat is encouraged. The greatest opportunity for fat burning is when you fast for 18 to 24 hours. There is also an increase in metabolic rate, leading up to the 18 or 24-hour mark, and then a decrease gradually. To keep the muscles from being broken down for energy the body produces a growth hormone that protects them and also encourages more burning of fat.

Within the liver, ketones are produced from the fat to create fuel for the body. The brain senses the increase in ketones and signals for these to be used for energy. After approximately 36 hours of fasting, leptin levels are at the lowest. During this time the hormones from the thyroid, which increase directly after fasting, begin to decline. Because of the need for fats to be moved around the body HDL, or high-density lipoprotein, and overall cholesterol increase. IGF, or insulin-like growth, declines. Mood is also enhanced because of new nerve growth.

These are changes anyone can expect on the first day or so of fasting. This is different for every person, but in general, these results can be expected. When a body becomes adapted to fasting, these above benefits will happen more efficiently, and even more health benefits can be expected.

When you become more adjusted to fasting abdominal or visceral fat is decreased. This is because the fat stored around the internal organs is being used for energy. Health benefits, such as lowering diabetes and cardiovascular disease risks, are a result of lowered resistance to insulin. Asthma and other inflammatory issues can be improved and preventing cellular growth can starve cancer cells.

Psychological Changes

Fasting also promotes many psychological changes in addition to the physical benefits. The mental strength required to commit and stick to fasting can be empowering and stress relieving. It can also break the emotional bond between eating and emotions. It can also help control your understanding of the hungry feeling. You learn to identify if you are truly hungry or desire something else. In addition, the feeling of hunger no longer triggers an immediate need for food, sometimes allowing this impulse to subside. Old habits slowly begin to be erased.

We are conditioned at a young age to turn to food for comfort. The severity and reasons may vary from person to person, but in general, when we become upset as babies, we are given food to help calm us. Different factors during your growth and develop influence your relationship with food. For example, sweets may have been given to you as a reward and restricted as a punishment when you were growing up. As you aged, you began to reward or deny yourself these same types of threats, strengthening this bond between these emotions and that food. Fasting forces you to experience those feelings without coping with them with food. Over time this deteriorates the association.

Top 10 Health Benefits for the Body

1. Changes to the role of hormones, cells, and genes. HGH, or human growth hormone, increases dramatically, cells repair, molecules and genes change to fight against the disease, and insulin lowers.

2. Loss of abdominal fat and overall weight. Ideally, you will eat fewer calories overall. This means if you continue or increase your daily activity you will lose weight. In addition, hormones being released also stimulate fat burning and overall weight loss. Finally, metabolism also increases during intermittent fasting. The combination of these three changes all increases the likelihood of losing weight.

3. Type 2 Diabetes risks reduced. Having high blood sugar increases the risk of developing type 2 diabetes. Fasting lowers the blood's glucose levels and insulin resistance. A side effect of type 2 diabetes, kidney damage, can also be avoided with intermittent fasting. This means that those at risk of developing diabetes and those who are currently suffering from type 2 diabetes can see improvement.

4. Lower inflammation and oxidative stress. Several chronic diseases are the result of oxidative stress in the body. Free radicals from oxidative stress are molecules that are unstable and react with molecules, like DNA, and hurt them. Inflammation is another cause of chronic diseases and fasting can reduce this negative driver.

5. Improved cardiovascular health. Risk factors associated with the world's number one killer can be improved with

intermittent fasting. Things like blood sugar levels, blood pressure, cholesterol, and triglycerides are all impacted.

6. Repairing cells is induced. During intermittent fasting autophagy or removal of waste is initiated at the cellular level. The cells are broken apart and the dysfunctional pieces are released. This process can help the body fight diseases such as Alzheimer's or cancer.

7. Cancer can be prevented. Cancer causes an increased cell growth. Fasting can slow the growth of cells, ultimately slowing the growth of cancer. In addition, chemotherapy's negative side effects can also be improved with intermittent fasting.

8. Brain health is improved. Brain function can be improved because of nerve cells have new growth. Brain problems, like depression, can also be improved because of BDNF, or brain-derived neurotrophic factor. If you have a risk of stroke, the potential damage to the brain can be prevented.

9. Alzheimer's disease can be prevented. This neurodegenerative disease does not have a cure. This means prevention if the best treatment. Intermittent fasting has been shown to prevent and minimize the severity of the disease. This prevention can also be effective with other neurodegenerative diseases like Huntington's and Parkinson's.

10. You can live longer. Animal studies have shown an increase in lifespan up to 83%. Part of this can be related

to the prevention of various diseases and increase in metabolism.

Chapter 3: Intermittent Fasting Benefits

Chances are, the reason you chose this book on intermittent fasting was to lose weight, but there are so many more additional benefits to following this lifestyle. The great news is that you are already fasting to some extent, while you are sleeping, so your body will know what to do. This means, whether you choose to fast for health or spiritual or weight control reasons, you can get more out of your experience understanding all the benefits this lifestyle offers.

Did you know, in addition to losing and controlling weight, you help your body regulate glucose? This means, for those that are diabetic or pre-diabetic, this form of fasting can help manage your disease without medical intervention. Also, you are jumpstarting your metabolism, helping you live longer (probably), and boosting your immune system. There are a lot of psychological and brain benefits as well. Because this is a lifestyle and not a "fad" or "crash" diet, you will see more long-lasting and compounded benefits over time, like losing and keeping that weight off. What it all boils down to is that almost every part of your body is improved through intermittent fasting. Below is a breakdown of some of the major health benefits that are known or are currently being studied that have shown promise.

Benefit #1: Lose Weight

Our bodies are programmed to store food as fat for energy when our food sources are low. When your ancestors were hunting and gathering, this was critical to survival. The more you could store up, the longer you could go between eating. Now, with the abundance and security of food, this is not necessary to your modern-day survival. Now, this stored fat just sits there, getting more and more fed, adding more and more weight.

When you do intermittent fasting, your body stops using the fuel coming in, the food and begins dipping into those internal storage pockets, your fat sources. The more that it dips into those stores, the more weight you lose from fat deposits. It also means this is a steady and natural way for your body to lose weight. It is biologically programmed to burn fat off. And because this is a sustainable lifestyle, it means you will continue to burn off fat and keep it off. Add benefit: you will see weight loss almost immediately!

Benefits #2: Stabilize Glucose

A diabetic is constantly thinking about their blood sugar levels or glucose. Most traditional treatment involves insulin injections or other medications. Instead of having to stabilize your glucose through medication, fasting can be a great alternative. It is also shown to improve the diabetic condition over time. For example, it can decrease the variability of glucose in your body throughout the day. One the amazing side effect of fasting is that it regulates how your body handles glucose and it increases your sensitivity to insulin.

When you are insensitive to insulin or you are resistant to its effects it means that too much glucose has accumulated in fat stored in tissues. During the fasting process, the body burns up the fat stores, making the accumulated glucose lower and lower, allowing the body, specifically the liver and muscles, become more sensitive or responsive to insulin. This is a great alternative to those looking to wean off medications or at least minimize the need for them.

Benefit #3: Live Longer

There are some studies out there that identify intermittent fasting as a means to a longer life. While all of these studies are conducted on animals, and there are not many published on the topic, it is uncertain how valid this is for humans, but it is possible. Scientists at the University of Chicago have made the connection that delaying or preventing illnesses that lead to death is possible through intermittent fasting, implying that people who do this will have healthier and longer lives. This is compared to those that eat the traditional 3 daily meals or just try to cut calories.

Another scientist, Mark Mattson, National Institute on Aging's head of the neuroscience lab, explains this even further. In his research, he has found that continually pushing your body with this mild stress makes it protect itself from damage to molecules by upping the cellular defense of the body. Also, the intermittent fasting processes help the body repair and maintain tissues by the constant stimulation. Your body is naturally fighting the aging process and is supporting each cell and organ to function efficiently and effectively.

Benefit #4: Immune System Improved

If you are looking to completely overhaul your immune system, there is good news. Your immune system can be completely regenerated through fasting, according to the findings at the University of Southern California. This is possible because of the new white blood cell production. These cells are responsible for fighting off infections. New cells created for the immune system replace the inefficient, damaged or just plain, old cells of the immune system during an intermittent fast.

For patients going through chemotherapy for cancer, research has shown that intermittent fasting, even for as little as one fast lasting 72 hours, could help protect the body from the negative side effects of the treatment. This cancer treatment is known for wreaking havoc on the immune system, but this may be a way to help support the system naturally. This could also help aged individuals who struggle with a compromised immune system. There are limited studies on this topic, but it does show promise!

Benefit #5: Stimulates Autophagy

Internal problems, such as organisms that are invading or pathogens, and external sources, such as a lack of vital nutrients, cause the body's cells to become stressed. Autophagy works to combat this and help the cells rebound from the stress. When a fast begins, your body begins the autophagy process. Your body begins to eliminate the build-up of damaged and dysfunctional proteins that are in cells. This buildup happens over time, but it is important that you get rid of this waste and begin to repair the cellular structure. There is limited research published that does suggest that this process that is stimulated during intermittent fasting can help your body fight off illnesses like Alzheimer's and cancer.

Benefit #6: Heal and Recover Faster

Some people turn to intermittent fasting to help with training for competitions or events like triathlons or marathons. For exercise enthusiasts, doing a fast overnight or for a day or two can be a good preparation for an intense work out on a non-fasting day. The research has found that performance is not impacted negatively but the recovery is improved. The combination of fasting and exercise requires monitoring; however, the benefits can be worth it for those looking for a better workout.

Additional research has also shown the bodybuilders or those weight training had increased muscle development when they trained after fasting. Although there is not a lot of research on this topic nor is what available conclusive, the proven improvement in sleep patterns and internal healing properties of fasting obviously aid the body in workout recovery.

Benefit #7: Ramp Up Metabolism

You will boost your metabolism when you restrict eating and then begin again. This is one of the major reasons you will lose weight and why so many people are thrilled about the re-discovery of this lifestyle. Some studies have reported the metabolism increasing by 14% during a short-term intermittent fast. Yes, long fasts will eventually lower metabolism; however, doing a short-term fast up to 60 hours can ramp up your metabolism.

This is also a distinctive feature of this lifestyle. Compared to a reduced calorie diet, intermittent fasting is sustainable and supporting. Calorie reduction actually is proven to hurt metabolism. Calorie reduction makes your body turn to muscles to burn for weight loss. The tissue of the muscles is used to break down calories. Because your body loses muscle it struggles to maintain a good metabolism. Intermittent fasting preserves the muscles and helps the immune system function seamlessly.

Benefit #8: Cancer Prevention

Several forms of cancer can be prevented by the production of the growth hormone that is stimulated during intermittent fasting. Cancer cells develop rapidly when the body continues to develop new cells. New cells are constantly developed when you are eating constantly. Take a break from eating, and your body has time to pause in the new-cell production process. This also allows the cells to form more naturally and not become cancerous.

Another cancer-fighting benefit is that intermittent fasting paired with chemotherapy or other cancer treatments can actually lessen the negative side effects and improve the outcomes of medical treatment. For example, breast cancer and skin cancer patients have seen an improved immune system that more effectively fights the cancerous cells when they followed an intermittent fasting diet during treatment. This is because the body supports the immune system and breaks down the "wall" that is preventing your immune system from doing its job against cancer.

Benefit #9: Prevent Chronic Disease

Another way that intermittent fasting can prevent cancer or chronic diseases is through reducing oxidative stress. This stress is a result of the production of reactive oxygen and antioxidant defense in the body becomes unbalanced. Free radicals, or molecules that are unstable and cause this imbalance, damage your body's DNA and protein. When you lose weight, you are automatically lowering your oxidative stress. When you lose it through intermittent fasting you are supporting your body to lower it even further. If you are looking to not only lose weight but also improve your well-being and overall health, this benefit should not be overlooked. The increase in antioxidant abilities is a major advantage of intermittent fasting.

Benefit #10: Improve your Skin

Cutting out dairy and staying away from processed foods are well-known cures for acne sufferers. Diet is the best way to control how your skin looks. Then it should come as no surprise that intermittent fasting will helps skin appear more radiant and clear.

Inflammation and acne are often symptoms of a food sensitivity or allergy. To determine if this is true for you, try adding some of the more common sensitivity foods back into your diet, one at a time. If or when you notice a change in your skin, you will have identified a trigger food that you know you can now avoid for a more glowing complexion (without the oil or red bumps).

The benefit does not stop at the skin. It is also shown to improve your hair and nails as well. Intermittent fasting helps both grow faster and remain healthier longer. This means that intermittent fasting does not just make you feel better, but it also helps you look better, too!

Benefit #11: Keep Your Heart Pumping

Your heart's function is probably one of the best reasons to lose excess weight. Lowering your body fat percentage has many benefits, but this particular one is vital to your immediate longevity. Lower weight means less kidney stress, reduced blood pressure, and more growth hormones produced. It also lowers your triglycerides and overall cholesterol levels. This is because the body is using it now for energy. All of these amazing benefits help boost your cardiovascular function.

The studies on the Mormon populations reveal that they tend to have better heart health. This is probably from the mixture of healthy lifestyle habits, such as avoiding drinks with caffeine or alcohol, smoking, and copious amounts of meat. In addition, intermittent fasting is a part of their religious practice. This is further evidence that making positive choices about your lifestyle and diet can lead to improved health in many areas, including your heart.

Benefit #12: Use Your Brain

In 2015 there was a study publicized at the Society for Neuroscience's meeting. The revelation shared was that your brain's health was significantly impacted in a positive manner by intermittent fasting. The study highlighted the results of the participants, which were both animal and human, and how the brain was stimulated in numerous distinctive ways. For example, memory was improved, recovery after an injury to the brain or stroke was enhanced, and neurons grew.

Those suffering from neurodegenerative diseases can see relief through intermittent fasting and also experience improved brain function. For those at risk or worried about developing a disease like Alzheimer's or Parkinson's, intermittent fasting can also lower the risk of developing them in the first place.

Benefit #13: Read Your Signals

Your body is constantly signaling or telling you what is going on inside. You should learn how to read the signals from your body and intermittent fasting to learn your body's hunger cues is a great tool. The psychological desire for food is the result of your body indicating to the brain that it is hungry. This happens before your body begins to starve so you can prevent it. The problem is that your body can become out of tune with true hunger versus the "normal" time of day that you eat. This is your mind and body playing tricks on you. Over time, through intermittent fasting, you will learn how to tell the difference between emotional or time-related "hunger" and true hunger. You will also notice how your body feels as it releases the toxins built up from processed foods, which may encourage you not to eat them again.

Another benefit to understanding your hunger is that you will learn not to take food for granted. The process of eating will become more enjoyable and pleasant. It will feel wrong to rush such a vital and pleasurable experience. This is heightened because you will have experienced what "real" hunger feels like. Sometimes this gratification is the only benefit you need to keep going!

Benefit #14: Set Routine

Getting your body into the swing of things occurs when you reprogram it to a new set of eating rules. Once you adjust to this new way of doing things your body will adjust its cues. You will stop feeling hungry at your past breakfast, lunch, dinner times. You will also notice your sleep improves. Creating this routine can be challenging, especially if you have a family or a demanding work schedule, but once you set one in place you will discover how beneficial it is to your health and life.

Benefit #15: Get in Touch with Your Spirit

Religions use fasting for a reason; it helps you get in touch with your higher power. Virtually every religion practices fasting in some form. Because of this, it should not surprise you to learn that having a deeper, spiritual connection and experience is normal when fasting. Feelings of peace or contentment are commonly associated with a fasting state. Moods can be regulated because of the reduction of stress and anxiety. Many therapists prescribe intermittent fasting as a treatment for mental, sexual, and emotional issues.

Another spiritual connection will be to the world around you and nature. You will have a clearer mind and become more positive. This could be from the empowerment of successfully completing a fasting day, the joy of watching the scale drop lower and lower, or the improvement in your overall health and appearance. Whatever the reason, make sure to enjoy this lovely benefit.

Chapter 4:
Fasting and Fat Burning and Satiation

There is a rumor circulating that the more you eat, the less hungry you will feel. This means you should eat smaller meals or snacks throughout the day, sometimes as often as 7 times in a day. The concept sounds plausible. If you never truly feel "hungry" because you are constantly eating than the choices, you make regarding what types of food you eat will be better and the amount of food consumed will be lower. Unfortunately, this is not true. Once our body begins a process that is necessary to its survival, like removing waste or drinking water or eating food, it needs to continue until the brain feels satisfied.

Another rumor is that reducing calories or controlling portions can help stop hunger pangs and make you lose weight. While you will most likely lose weight, you will remain hungry. This is because the hormones that tell your brain that it is full and satisfied or still hungry did not get enough juice to balance out. This type of diet is unsustainable for many people, because of these hunger pangs, which results in them losing back all and sometimes more weight than before. It is unsustainable because our bodies are programmed to survive. Hunger is needed for this survival. This means that if it feels that it is always hungry, the hunger triggers will get more and more intense until you finally give in.

This leaves the challenge of how to lose weight and not be hungry all the time. The answer has been in front of us for as long as humanity has been around: fasting.

Fasting removes food from the forefront of your mind and also front-loads your food intake. In addition, it changes your eating schedule so ghrelin, the hunger hormone, is released at different times. Of course, this takes time for your body to adjust, but once it does, the body feels less hungry and is losing weight.

Food at the Front

Eating too many calories will result in weight gain, as evidenced again and again in research, but drastically cutting calories back at meals has been shown to be ineffective at losing weight and keeping it off. This means that on non-fasting days it is important to try to maintain a healthy intake of calories, not gorging yourself on food, but not holding back at breakfast, lunch, and dinner. Those people that eat a standard number of calories on a non-fast day show more satisfaction and less hunger than those that overeat or that try to cut calories back.

When the body feels more satisfied it has balanced itself with the hunger signals, making the hunger survival instinct happy. This means you will lose weight and be able to keep it off. It also means that on fasting days you will begin to feel less hungry as well. After all, as seen above, not eating is better for our instinctual wiring than eating small amounts.

Timing is critical to your body's metabolism. Research continues to be published that shows, when you eat, is almost as important as what is eaten. Our bodies typically function on a 24-hour clock naturally, triggered by light and dark, but as you have probably discovered for yourself, you can adjust your behavioral, physical, and mental responses depending on your needed schedule or the changes in daylight throughout the year. For example, if you change jobs and no longer are able to eat lunch at 12 PM and instead need to eat it at 2 PM, your body will feel hungry for a few days at noon but after a while, you will be re-programmed to feel hungry at 2 PM and not 12. The wiring for our rhythms that are based on light, such as sleeping, are more difficult to re-program, but those do not have much to do with hunger. Hunger can be a 24-hour sensation.

As your body goes through it daily flow, hormones and enzymes are released in anticipation of certain activities and transporters of glucose are varied. All of this affects how the body burns energy and loses fat. These responses control your weight, blood sugar, cholesterol, and many other important systems in the body.

Riding the Waves

It has been proven that the hunger hormone is lowest when you first wake up. This is why you may be like many other people and need to wait a bit to eat breakfast. But have you stopped to think about why this is true? Your body has just gone through possibly the longest stretch of time without eating. It would make sense that you would be ravenous when waking, but instead, the body seems satisfied. This is because the body is used to this rhythm and produces less of the hunger hormone.

Next, the body anticipates your schedule. When it senses that it is almost your breakfast, lunch or dinnertime, it releases ghrelin, the hunger hormone. But here is the really interesting thing; the body does not keep producing ghrelin until you eat something. After a bit, the hormone dissipates, regardless of food consumed. It takes about 2 hours for your body to stop responding to the hunger hormone that was released in anticipation of a meal. Think about when you became too busy to eat at your normal time. Did your body eventually "forget" it was hungry? Or did the hunger never even present itself? This is because of the "waves" of hormones being released and then subsiding.

Research has shown that throughout a 24-hour day, fasting or non-fasting, ghrelin is released at the same levels. This means that you are not hungrier on fasting days, but rather you are the same. This means that as your body becomes conditioned to eating on a different schedule, you will become less hungry, not more. When you are less hungry, you are less likely to eat more, and less likely to gain weight. But you are more likely to lose it!

Women do show a markedly more intense and faster change to ghrelin during a fasting state. This means women will adjust faster to a new eating pattern than men. To account for this, women may be more suitable to do a one-on-one-off fast while men may benefit from a three-on-four-off type of fast to see similar results. When you fast, whether you are a man or woman, you can expect your ghrelin levels to drop. You can expect your body to send you messages that you are less hungry and more satisfied. You can also expect to not be "able" or do not desire to eat as much as you used to. You will feel fuller faster. You may also no longer crave the treats you used to turn to on a regular basis. This demonstrates the biological and mental changes happening in your body.

Overall, this means that fasting can and does make you feel less hungry and lose weight after your body adjusts to the new rhythm. Your body will adjust the release of ghrelin when you train it to and you can ride out the waves of hunger as they pass without turning into a ravenous animal. Fasting is truly one of the most sustainable and effective methods for losing and keeping weight off!

Chapter 5:
The Science of Hunger

Inside your brain, there is a pathway that is programmed for your love of food, specifically the really "good" foods. This pathway is not something you were born with, but it was developed over time. The neurochemical, sensory and metabolic reactions fired the minute you tasted that first "treat." The pleasure center in your brain, the mesolimbic area, is what became engaged. Digestive acids were secreted when your stomach received the signal from the vagus nerve. Insulin began being pumped out by the pancreas. The increase in sugar, fat, and starch are accommodated by increased liver production. During this whole process, your brain simply remembers that whatever it was that you just ate was good. This begins a lasting impression of that particular food.

Your relationship with food as a human is difficult. Many of your body's systems occur automatically, such as your endocrine, circulatory, and respiratory systems. Eating is distinctive because it is completely voluntary and critical to your life. This is the reason for the intense desire for food that you feel. This is a problem now because, instead of the age-old problem of not having enough to eat, we now face the issue of having too much. Your body is not programmed to handle the unrestrained options that are available to your uncontrolled appetite.

Our appetite often drives our behavior, so it is important to learn how to control it. This control has been difficult to pinpoint because it is an incredibly complex process. All the senses, the chemistry of the brain and gut, and even psychology are involved. This is what science is still working to understand. Part of this research includes looking to the past to decipher how our ancestors controlled their hunger and how we can use this to our advantage. Fasting is part of this research.

For your ancestors, the state of your weight is what they sought after. These ancestors did not know where their next meal was coming from and often faced dangerous risks while trying to get something to eat. For example, sampling crops that they did not know or hunting animals for meat endangered their lives almost daily. This means that when they did have good food they needed to eat as much as possible. Human bodies are programmed to eat a lot when it is available and especially eat fat-filled food. There is a reason your body takes several minutes to recognize that it is full after eating a meal. After 20 minutes your body will recognize it is still hungry, full, or over full. This served your ancestors well because they could eat a lot before their body shut them off, but it is not so helpful now.

Your body does work internally to regulate itself. Your eating habits are established through your routine. When you consume meals or snacks at certain times of the day on a regular basis your body begins to anticipate eating and sends a hunger signal through a hormone named ghrelin. This hormone is created in the gut and is produced by our dietary schedule and even possibly the smell or sight of food. It creates the sensation of an empty stomach that the brain interprets as feeling hungry. In the brain, the hypothalamus, which is the director of the metabolism, the midbrain's mesolimbic center, which is the pleasure center, and the hindbrain, which governs unconscious procedures, are all hit by the production of ghrelin. This is why the brain listens to the signal from the gut.

There is a balance to the production of ghrelin and the signal it sends to the brain. This counter-balance begins in the upper intestine and stomach. This is a physical response to becoming full. The tension and stretching of the organs send a signal after time to the brain. This sensation includes three more items that signal the brain. CCK, or cholecystokinin, is a peptide from the upper intestine. It tells the brain you are satisfied and to stop eating. This only lasts a short time compared to ghrelin. What arrives in the brain after CCK are GLP-1 and PYY, hormones that reinforce the signal to stop. These hormones come from the lower gut and some of it stays behind to also talk to the stomach. These hormones let the stomach know it needs to pause sending food to the digestive tract until it has processed what is already there. GLP-1 also alerts the pancreas to send more insulin out to help absorb the sugar from the foods ingested and then store them in the fat for later energy.

If the balance between these two systems becomes off-kilter and you are still eating too much and gaining weight, there is another natural regulator: leptin. Your body's fat produces this hormone that stifles the appetite. The more the hormone is produced is proportional to the fat tissue in the body. Once the hormone hits the bloodstream, it travels to the brain's hypothalamus and seeks a partnership with neuropeptides that stimulate the appetite. This partnership results in the neuropeptides being slightly stifled. Ideally, this means that the more weight you have the more leptin you have to help control appetite.

The reason these internal forces do not always self-regulate your body is that there are approximately twenty-four other peptides and hormones that control the appetite. This means that changing just one or two hormones or levels will not result in a large change in appetite and weight. It truly does require a complete overhaul of the system.

Additional research into some of the complex receptors in the brain that create gateways for appetite signals is underway. MC-3 and MC-4 are the two currently most interesting pathways. MC-4 can malfunction, not allowing the "correct" signals to be interpreted in the brain, and MC-3 can also become dysfunctional and not allow the body to balance itself. Other research is being conducted regarding the "addiction" to eating and the chemical responses our brains and bodies go through when eating or abstaining.

Chapter 6:
Preparing for Intermittent Fasting

Be aware of how your body will most likely feel while doing a fast is important. These physical effects can derail you if you do not expect them. For the first couple of days, it is common for you to be uncomfortable but usually by the third day the feelings subside.

Part of the knowledge you need includes the health benefits and concerns. Fasting can reduce the risks of several diseases and minimize the effects of others. But some chronic health conditions may not be suitable for intermittent fasting or any other kind of fast. If you suffer from any health concern, it is important to talk with your doctor about what you want to do and be aware of what this new lifestyle can do for your health, both positive and negative. Conditions that may not be suitable for this diet include pregnancy, kidney issues, diabetes, immune system problems and cardiovascular irregularities.

Get Ready to Detox

Intermittent fasting refers to the time frame between fasting and non-fasting. This means a fast could last a few hours to a few days. It is important to decide and commit to a time frame that you want to try. This may require speaking with your doctors to find a suitable option for you, or at least for you to take a realistic inventory of where you are starting. If you have shown no control over eating patterns before, jumping in for a multi-day fast could set you up for failure. Choose to start small and ramp up as you experience more success and control. To help with this decision process, determine exactly what you want to achieve. Be clear with yourself. Set the commitment by telling someone what you are going to do and why you are doing. Enlist them to help keep you on track. Get a journal and write down why you are making this lifestyle change. Use this journal every day to write about your fasting, even before you begin. Keep track of your thoughts and feelings on what you are about to embark on. Continue writing during your fasting to chronicle your changes and the process. This will help you when you are feeling low. You can look back and see all the progress you have already made!

Your body is going to go through some pretty amazing changes when you make this switch. Part of that process will be a "detox" from the chemical build up in your body. This means it may make you feel sick, weak, or tired. You may also have headaches or diarrhea. If you can, consider taking time off from work to help with this transition, or at least find ways throughout the day to rest and ride out these side effects. If you want to try to lessen these side effects of the detox, try cutting back on toxic habits a few weeks before the fast. This means pulling back or stopping drinking alcohol or smoking. Caffeine is another one. If you do not want to experience the harshest withdrawal symptoms, start cutting back about two weeks before you want to start your fast. You should also change up your diet a couple of weeks before the fast. Foods like refined sugar or carbohydrates can deposit toxins in your body that it will need to detox during the fast. Cutting back these before the fast will help minimize the symptoms of withdrawal. You are allowing your body to slowly start getting rid of the toxins before the big push during the fast.

Changing your habits and diet can be hard. If you want to start a few weeks before you begin intermittent fasting, set a goal to eliminate or cut back on one item per day. For example, cut back from 5 cigarettes to 2. Only have 1 glass of wine with dinner instead of 2. Begin minimizing dairy and meat products in your daily diet. Focus on eating more vegetables. Making these changes a little at a time will help the body adjust to the changes during the fast making it a much more pleasant experience.

As you approach the date of your fast, cut back your diet even further. About 2 days before you want to begin, try eating only fruits and vegetables. Dairy and meats are harder on the body to digest and rid the body of toxins. Also, up your fluid intake. Drink a lot of water, fruit juice or tea. Make sure to drink fresh and natural fruit juice with no added sugar or chemicals.

It is normal to experience fatigue or being tired during the preparation since your body is going through a mini detox. This means that you should change your exercise routine up a little bit. If you are used to doing more aggressive exercises, consider cutting them back to more moderate or gentle choices. For those that are not in the habit of exercising, increase your activity levels a few weeks before the fasting date to get your vascular system and lymphatic fluids pumping. Also, because you are probably feeling tired, it is important to honor the body and get more rest. Getting plenty of sleep and rest will determine how successful you are in your fast. This means getting adequate sleep at night and being mindful of your activity during the day. It is a wise idea to time the beginning of your fast when your schedule is not as busy, so you can prioritize this part of the process. It is one of the largest indicators of your success!

10 Do's and Don'ts

1. Do know your role. If you are battling a health condition and should not fast, do not change to this lifestyle. Sometimes these conditions are temporary, like pregnancy, and you can begin your fast at a later time, but some conditions are continual.

2. Don't forget to include your healthcare professional. Even if you do not have a health concern or previous condition, it is a good idea to check in with your doctor before you start. This way you have someone who knows what you are doing and can help you monitor your health, not just your weight.

3. Do consider your lifestyle. Choose to start fasting during a low-stress time or when there is a lull in your social calendar. Trying to start a major change like intermittent fasting during the holidays, for example, is a set up for failure. Instead, choose to integrate this into your life in the spring or summer when your stress levels and exertion is lower. This can be applied to your week as well. Choose the days of the week that you will be fasting according to your typical schedule. If you find Monday's require more physical exertion or have more stress, consider setting that day as a non-fast day. Some people like to fast on the weekend when they can rest and have less going on while

others like to fast during the week, so they can enjoy on the weekends. Choose what works for you.

4. To avoid the "last supper syndrome" or the "victory feast." Do not gorge yourself the night or day before a fasting day. Focus on a healthy, balanced meal instead of loading up on calories and junk foods. This will not only make you feel better that night but will let your body switch modes easier when it begins fasting. The same thing goes for the day after a fasting period.

5. Do get your house as prepared as your mind. Clear out your kitchen of temptation. Toss foods and drinks that you crave and replace them with healthier options that you can enjoy when you are done with your fasting day or days.

6. Do stay alert of your changes. Discomfort is normal, especially when you are starting intermittent fasting. But you need to be in tune with your body. Feelings of dizziness, muscle weakness (not just tiredness), and heart palpitations are all conditions that indicate you need to stop immediately. This may indicate that you need more time to ease into the type of fast you want or there is a medical reason you should not be fasting. Whatever the case, listen and obey the major signals of your body and stay in contact with your doctor if something like this occurs.

7. Don't ramp up the exercise routine. While fasting, especially in the beginning, do not try to push your physical exertion too hard. Even if you are used to high-intensity workouts, your body may not be ready to tackle

that and tackle a fast. Things like gentle yoga can be more beneficial for your body than a cardio class.

8. Do take supplements. Many of the necessary vitamins can be found in supplements. Liquids can be easier for digestion than pills or chews. A good multivitamin can help your body get the vitamins it needs without the additional calories. Since you are also consulting your physician during this process, discussing your vitamin needs is also an important part of the prep process.

9. Don't forget about water. There is a significant amount of water in foods that we eat so it is important to replace that with straight water when we are not eating food. To tell if you are getting enough water, check the color when you pee. If the color is a very pale yellow, you are getting enough hydration. Anything darker and you need to up your H2O intake.

10. Don't forget to have fun! Escape those cravings and the pangs of hunger by treating yourself to something you enjoy. Get a massage, treat yourself to a manicure, or dream about how you will look in that hot outfit while you are window-shopping. Choose activities that keep you away from food, especially if you are trying to avoid the hunger signals. Also, consider removing or un-following social media accounts that are food-focused.

Chapter 7:
Scientific Methods of Intermittent Fasting

Ideas, like eating every other day or skipping a meal per day, are all ideas of intermittent fasting. Diet enthusiasts and exercise fanatics post these concepts on blogs and websites and even publish books about them. There are many ways you can transition to intermittent fasting; some of the more popular are outlined here.

It is important to preface that most of the approaches to intermittent fasting here are based on various scientific studies. Many of these studies used animals for participants and most of the human studies were on participants with a particular condition, like diabetes or obesity, or a parameter, such as religion. If you are a healthy adult looking to participate in intermittent fasting, there are few studies conducted on your parameters. There are several studies being conducted currently that seek to support the animal studies and different effects on various body compositions. Until then, the currently published studies will be used for evidence here.

There are several similarities in the various approaches to intermittent fasting. One major similarity amongst them all is the realization of true hunger versus a craving. It breaks the link between "hunger" and "desire" or "panic" and realigns it with "power," "pride," or "success" (Ganley, 1989). Also, any type of intermittent fast being followed will require time for adjustment. Most people will need anywhere from 3 to 6 weeks to adjust to the new habits (Longo, Mattson, 2014). While the body goes through this adjustment period, it is normal for you to feel uncomfortable. You will probably be irritable, tired, and weak (Johnstone 2007). After the body adjusts in a few weeks, the "pain" of being hungry and the "bad" mood should improve (Wing et al. 1991).

It is also important that, no matter the kind of intermittent fast you choose, that you also focus on eating nutritional meals on your non-fasting days. Things like minerals, vitamins, protein, fat, and fiber are all nutrients that need to be consumed for optimal health. Since they are not taken in on fasting days, ensuring that your body receives what it needs on non-fasting days is important for weight loss and keeping your body healthy. Also, hydration is important. Water is necessary for life and is especially important for any form of intermittent fast. Not only does drinking water on fasting days help you stay hydrated, it also helps you pass through hunger feelings easier. Some recommendations include sipping on various beverages during fasting days, including bone broth, but it is uncertain how this affects the overall level of energy, appetite, or the ultimate outcome of the fast.

Now that you are aware of the similarities between all types of intermittent fasts, let us explore the different kinds you should consider.

Fasting on alternate days

For every two days, food is restricted for 24 hours and then consumed for 24 hours. Water is allowed on fasting and non-fasting days. This type of fast is the most common one people refer to in publications and also is the most researched form of intermittent fasting on animals. Few studies with this eating pattern and humans have been published to date. The longevity of the animals in the studies was the primary purpose of the research. Several factors were found to affect the outcome of the results, such as age, breed, and exercise (Longo & Mattson, 2014).

One of the human studies that shadowed men and women eating for 24 hours and then fasting for 24 hours concluded that participants lost about 4% of their fat mass over 21 days on this diet. Overall participants lost about 2½% of their overall body weight in that time. In addition, the insulin sensitivity of all participants increased (Heilbronn, Civitarese, et al. 2005). The animal-study counterparts to this study indicate that this form of intermittent fasting does also help your body respond to stress better. Heilbronn and Civitarese's research is the first study in humans that also supports this find.

Tips for alternate day fasting:

- On a fasting day:

    √ Always keep water by your side.

    √ Enlist your friends and family to help you stay motivated. Let them know that you are trying something new and ask them to be supportive and encouraging.

√ If you break down and break your fast, make it into a non-fast day and eat normally. Follow your same schedule of fast and non-fast days starting the next day.

- On a non-fasting day:

  √ Eat a lot of protein, especially at lunch and dinner. This will make you feel more satisfied on your fasting days.

  √ Do not try to cut down calories or skip meals. Enjoy your food! And eat all your daily calories.

Example weekly plan:

- Sunday: begin eating at 8 AM and eat normally throughout the day, exercise intensely

- Monday: stop eating at 8 AM and begin fasting, exercise lightly or moderately

- Tuesday: begin eating at 8 AM and eat normally throughout the day, exercise intensely

- Wednesday: stop eating at 8 AM and begin fasting, exercise lightly or moderately

- Thursday: begin eating at 8 AM and eat normally throughout the day, exercise intensely

- Friday: stop eating at 8 AM and begin fasting, exercise lightly or moderately

- Saturday: begin eating at 8 AM and eat normally throughout the day, exercise intensely

Fasting Trial

If even the concept of starting an alternate day fast or any intermittent fast is frightening, consider this regimen. It is just simply a singular attempt at fasting. No commitment beyond one day. Ideally, you would forgo food for a full 24 hours, but you could decide to try it for less or more, depending on your preference. This trial allows you to feel what it is like to be intentionally hungry and how to get used to it. Once you make it past your original fasting window you can then try another version of intermittent fasting if you want. It is important to remember that some of the feelings during a short-term fast are normal and should not be used as a reason to not fast further. In reality, it is even more reason to do it! These side effects are signals that your body needs to get rid of toxins.

Tips for a fasting trial:

- Drink tea to help make the time pass easier.

- Watch your body signals for indications that it is going into too much stress. These signals can be extreme mood swings, heart palpitations or lethargy are signs you may need to break your fast.

Example weekly plan:

- Sunday: eat normally

- Monday: eat normally

- Tuesday: eat normally until 6 PM

- Wednesday: do not eat until 6 PM, eat a large but reasonable meal

- Thursday: eat normally

- Friday: eat normally

- Saturday: eat normally

"LeanGains"

The nutritional writer and personal trainer from Sweden, Martin Berkhan, was the biggest promoter of this intermittent fasting plan. In this daily fasting plan, the participant spends 16 hours a day fasting and then eats 3 traditional meals in 8 hours. For example, you would fast from 9 PM until 1 PM the following day. After 1 PM you would eat your daily caloric intake split into about 3 meals. The first meal should be packed with protein, especially if you exercise right before. Berkhan recommends that you schedule your workout right as your fast ends and before your first meal to optimize your metabolic burn. Another recommendation from Berkhan is to eat more fat and carbohydrates in the evening meal. Carbohydrates should be eaten on days you work out and fats on days you rest. While much of Berkhan's recommendations are helpful, there are some that are not scientifically reinforced. For example, he advises that you should take BCAA's or branched chain amino acids, about 10 minutes before a workout. This is to help preserve your muscles during the workout.

Studies conducted on men and women partaking in this form of intermittent fasting show there is a difference in gender response. For example, women see more success when their fasting window is smaller. Women who fasted for 14 hours instead of 16 saw better results. Men did well in the traditional 16-hour fasting plan.

In theory, this plan is plausible for health and weight loss. It does reprogram the hunger hormones to be released daily at a different time and impacts the metabolism. The challenge is that this form of intermittent fasting has very few scientific studies backing up the kind of fast.

Tips for LeanGains fasting:

- When you are fasting, keep drinking water. Staying hydrated will help you satiate hunger but also will keep you from becoming dehydrated as your body is cleansing itself of toxins.

- When you are beginning this fasting lifestyle, allow yourself to drink a very small amount of caffeine such as black coffee or tea, both with no sweeteners. This will both help you feel fuller and will also help with any detoxing headache. Stick to 1 cup of coffee or tea during your fasting hours.

- Keep busy during fasting hours. Keeping yourself busy will keep you from thinking about the hunger during fasting hours.

- When your fasting hours end be cautious of what you eat for your first meal. You do not want to gorge yourself. This is especially critical for weight loss. Consider limiting your first meal to only 3 foods and allowing yourself to eat as much as you like of those 3 foods. This way your body is not excited about new flavors and will signal you earlier that it is full.

Example weekly plan:

- Sunday: do not eat until 4 PM. Eat 1 average meal at 4 PM, then again at 6 PM and a third at 9 PM. Do not eat anything after 4 AM the latest.

- Monday: do not eat until 4 PM. Eat 1 average meal at 4 PM, then again at 6 PM and a third at 9 PM. Do not eat anything after 4 AM the latest.

- Tuesday: do not eat until 4 PM. Eat 1 average meal at 4 PM, then again at 6 PM and a third at 9 PM. Do not eat anything after 4 AM the latest.

- Wednesday: do not eat until 4 PM. Eat 1 average meal at 4 PM, then again at 6 PM and a third at 9 PM. Do not eat anything after 4 AM the latest.

- Thursday: do not eat until 4 PM. Eat 1 average meal at 4 PM, then again at 6 PM and a third at 9 PM. Do not eat anything after 4 AM the latest.

- Friday: do not eat until 4 PM. Eat 1 average meal at 4 PM, then again at 6 PM and a third at 9 PM. Do not eat anything after 4 AM the latest.

- Saturday: do not eat until 4 PM. Eat 1 average meal at 4 PM, then again at 6 PM and a third at 9 PM. Do not eat anything after 4 AM the latest.

The "Warrior" fast

Another daily fast, this is a hyped-up version of the "LeanGains." While LeanGains encourages eating several meals during the non-fasting window, the warrior diet recommends only 1 super meal, normally eaten around dinnertime. The reasoning used to explain this method is that it is aligned more closely with natural circadian rhythms. These rhythms are our natural response to day and night and the 24-hour cycle of life. This intermittent fasting plan is supposed to support the body while removing toxins and supporting our natural needs. These claims; however, do not have scientific backing.

In a study conducted on average-weight human participants, those that ate only one meal per day, instead of 3 meals with the same overall calories, saw more positive results. Those that ate their caloric intake in one meal lost more overall body weight and retained more lean body mass or muscle mass. This study lasted for 8 weeks. The challenge with this method of intermittent fasting is the hunger hormone. In this study, participants experienced an increase in hunger signals (Stote *et al.*, 2007). This suggests that the hormones controlling your appetite will not adjust. More research is needed to support these findings and assess the claims above.

Tips for Warrior fasting:

- Work into it. This is not a lifestyle for someone who has not had luck with changing their diet before or have been following another diet plan like high-carbohydrates. Consider starting with a lesser intense version and work up to this intense intermittent fasting plan.

- Start and stay positive. Beginning this type of intermittent fast with the idea that it is terrible or that you will fail means you probably will. Instead, stay positive and remember that you can do this. Think of all the reasons you are doing it and why it is important you keep at it.

- Increase your electrolytes. Add sea salt to your water or eat food with a lot of potassium and magnesium. Your body excretes a lot of electrolytes in the detox process and should be replaced naturally.

Example weekly plan:

- Sunday: do not eat until 6 PM. Workout intensively and then eat 1 large meal around 7 PM. Stop eating by 2 AM at the latest.

- Monday: do not eat until 6 PM. Workout intensively and then eat 1 large meal around 7 PM. Stop eating by 2 AM at the latest.

- Tuesday: do not eat until 6 PM. Workout intensively and then eat 1 large meal around 7 PM. Stop eating by 2 AM at the latest.

- Wednesday: do not eat until 6 PM. Workout intensively and then eat 1 large meal around 7 PM. Stop eating by 2 AM at the latest.

- Thursday: do not eat until 6 PM. Workout intensively and then eat 1 large meal around 7 PM. Stop eating by 2 AM at the latest.

- Friday: do not eat until 6 PM. Workout intensively and then eat 1 large meal around 7 PM. Stop eating by 2 AM at the latest.

- Saturday: do not eat until 6 PM. Workout intensively and then eat 1 large meal around 7 PM. Stop eating by 2 AM at the latest.

Periodic fasting

While this is similar in theory to the alternate day fast, it is really just a longer version of the LeanGains method less frequently. The idea is that this fast lasts for 24 hours and normal eating can resume for another determined amount of time. Various people have advocated this intermittent fasting regimen because it can begin at any time and as often as you want. One of the most modern proponents includes Brad Pilon, author of *Eat Stop Eat*. He recommends doing this fast up to 5 times in a week. Dr. John Berardi's original article that introduced this concept stated that it should not be done more than twice a week.

Intermittent Fasting

Tips for periodic fasting:

- Consider what you eat on non-fasting days and choose wisely to maximize the potential weight loss and health benefits.

- Twenty-four hours can be a challenge to fast, but the good news is that if you time it well most of the time will be while sleeping. Using rest and busy awake hours can help the days of fasting move by easier.

Example weekly plan:

- Sunday: eat normally

- Monday: eat normally until 6 PM, being fasting at 6 PM

- Tuesday: do not eat until 6 PM, have one adequate meal for dinner to resume normal eating habits

- Wednesday: eat normally

- Thursday: eat normally until 6 PM, begin fasting at 6 PM

- Friday: do not eat until 6 PM, have one adequate meal for dinner to resume normal eating habits

- Saturday: eat normally

"Fat Loss Forever"

According to many of the published studies on both animals and humans, fasting up to 36 hours results in the most metabolic boost and fat burn. This is the basis of this intermittent fasting plan. Developed by Dan Go and John Romaniello, they recommend fasting for 36 hours, best observed on a busy day, then following a structured fasting lifestyle for the majority of the rest of the week. During this time, you should also be working out with weights and using your bodyweight. Many people enjoy this method of intermittent fasting because it also builds in a "cheat" day.

We all practice some form of intermittent fasting every day, because we have several hours that pass between mealtimes, and even more so overnight. The idea of Fat Loss Forever is to use that fasting time to your benefit. Despite the benefits associated with making smart choices about our fasting time and capitalizing on the knowledge of scientifically backed fasting time frames, it can be challenging to keep switching up the fasting and eating schedule every day during the week. Although the founders offer a calendar to follow this method, it can be confusing and not allow your body to make the necessary adjustments to a new eating schedule.

Tips for Fat Loss Forever fast:

- Follow the calendar and do not skip a day. This fast requires commitment and consistency.

- Do not follow this plan if you do not do well with "cheat" days or lose momentum quickly. Taking this day off can make it harder to go back in. In addition, gorging yourself will make the remaining days fasting, especially the 36 hours, more uncomfortable.

Example weekly plan:

- Sunday: eat normally until 9 PM

- Monday: no food intake, moderate exercise

- Tuesday: do not eat until 9 AM, eat healthy until 9 PM, weight lifting exercise

- Wednesday: begin eating normally at 9 AM, moderate exercise

- Thursday: do not monitor your eating habits, weight lifting exercise or high intensity

- Friday: Begin eating at 9 AM until 12 PM, begin fasting at 12 PM, moderate exercise

- Saturday: Begin eating at 9 AM until 12 PM, begin fasting at 12 PM, moderate exercise or rest day

Other Versions of Intermittent Fasting

Because of the lack of scientific research on human participants and various body compositions and health states, there is still not one version of intermittent fasting that is recommended more than another. In addition, this has opened the door for an almost unlimited variety of intermittent fasts.

The key indication that a fast you are looking to follow is an intermittent fast is that it has both a fasting and non-fasting period defined. People most often people will adopt different versions to fit their lifestyle and needs. Choose and tweak various intermittent fasting plans to make it successful for you.

Chapter 8:
Common Intermittent Myth's Busted

It is likely that the moment you decided to lose weight and focus on your nutritional health you were bombarded with all sorts of ideas of what a "good" diet and lifestyle looks like. This can come from anywhere and can be a curse more than a blessing. There is some validity in recommendations regarding different body types, but many of the common practices today are just myths. Many have scarce scientific credibility. Typically, it is half-truth and half-myth, developed from understudied or tested ideas. It is even worse when there is a study, but it is quoted out of context or misinterpreted.

These myths are prevalent because they continue to be spread. The more it is repeated the more people believe it. It means to us, psychologically, that it must be true and therefore does not require any further research. Otherwise, why would you hear about it all the time? Always consider the source of the information and do research for yourself. This means you have to do some digging, but when it comes to your health, it is worth it.

Another reason that common myths about fasting occur is the financial gain through the media. Companies want to sell more products to make more money. This means that they will encourage you to take action that will result in more of their products being used. Think of those toothpaste commercials. You only need a fraction of the amount they show on a toothbrush in the commercial. Or what would happen to cereal companies if you realized you do not need to eat all that food first thing in the morning? Constant snacking would require you to be constantly reaching for food, which you would probably reach for a nutritional bar or shake.

Finally, have you ever sat down to read a scientific study? It is hard. It takes time and focus if you can even understand the language being used. Most people need an academic background to get through a paper and even then, it is not guaranteed you could draw conclusions from their findings. This means that the majority of people rely on others to interpret the data, which may not always be accurate.

Fasting has been on the battering end of several health "experts" with claims that it will actually make you gain weight, lose muscle, damage your brain, destroy your metabolism and increase your hunger tenfold. Some of the top myths about intermittent fasting and where those myths originated need to be understood so you can learn what is true and what is a myth. This will allow you to make the most educated decision for yourself.

Top 5 Myths Debunked

1. *MYTH: Eat a big breakfast, a good-sized lunch, and a little bit of dinner.* This concept originated from the idea that eating later can cause weight gain. For example, snacking before bed causes an increase in weight. Studies that are quoted to support this myth include those of workers who work late night shifts and their body

composition and health. Keep in mind the context of this article. It is not controlled and is only observational on topics like lipids in the blood and tolerance of glucose. The truth is that having a healthier lifestyle, that does not involve late-night snacking, will keep your weight down more than pushing your entire caloric intake into one and a half meals.

The research that backs this up includes many studies done on Ramadan fasting. This religious practice involves fasting during daylight hours. At night it is customary to have a large meal. Such a practice has actually shown to improve body fat percentages in some examples! In most, it had a neutral effect. Another study tested two groups; one that ate most of their calories in the morning and another group that ate most at night. The group that ate more in the morning lost more muscle mass and retained more fat than the latter group.

2. *MYTH: Fasting makes you lose muscle and strength.* It is not unrealistic to think that eating a lot of calories before working out would give you more energy to burn, but the opposite is actually true. Several studies have been conducted on activity during fasting. Most of the negative side effects occur when you restrict fluids on a fasting day, otherwise, there is less impact on endurance or ability. In addition, muscle mass is more likely to be retained during intermittent fasting than other diet plans because the energy is coming from fat and not muscle mass. While training for competitions and races should not be done while fasting for increased nutritional needs, regular

exercise while fasting will not impact the results or your ideal body composition.

3. *MYTH: Cortisol increases.* When someone fasts for a long time or restricts calories drastically the body becomes stressed and the levels of cortisol rise. This is required because blood sugar is necessary, and cortisol helps regulate it. The challenge is that this occurs when the body is truly starving not when intermittently fasting. This little hormone is responsible for stabilizing the immune system, maintaining blood pressure, and reducing lipids, proteins, and glucose. Some increase in cortisol is important; it is what literally gets you out of bed in the morning. It also helps burn fat. It can also be increased by stress. Studies have shown that intermittent, short-term fasting does not affect cortisol levels. In participants that did see a small increase noticed other positive side effects like weight loss and maintained muscle mass.

4. *MYTH: Not eating breakfast makes you fat.* The studies that originate this myth are focused on a non-regulated pattern for eating. The participants that did not "eat" breakfast was reported as eating unhealthy food selections, like donuts and sugar-loaded drinks, on the run. Those that did sit down to a morning meal did indicate they had, overall, better dietary habits.

This lower regard for health is what causes weight gain in this scenario, just like having too large of a breakfast. The concern regarding insulin sensitivity is debunked by the fact that the time does not matter when glycogen is depleted. When you first wake in the morning your body has gone without glycogen for several hours, making the body more sensitive to insulin the next time you eat. This can happen for a meal at lunch-time or at dinner, depending on when your body uses up its glycogen stores.

5. *MYTH: Your body thinks you are starving when you fast.* The idea that when the body begins to starve your metabolic rate decreases is not related to intermittent fasting. Skipping a meal or going one or two days without eating does not make your body starve. Studies have shown, time and time again, that the metabolic rate is not lowered until the body has gone without any food for 60 to 96 hours. It depends on the person, but in general, not eating a meal or for an entire day will not decrease metabolism or make your body think it is starving. During the hours leading up to "starving" your metabolism actually ramps up! When a fast hit the 36 to 48-hour mark metabolism is at an all-time high, up to 10% higher than normal.

BONUS MYTH: Eat small meals often throughout the day. It is possible that this myth was born from the studies on appetite control and meal frequency, but it is important to note that these studies are limited. They are also not applicable to real-world scenarios. In addition, it is important to note, like the other myths, that just because there is a correlation between those that eat more frequently and weighing less does not mean that the meal frequency is the reason or cause of the weight. In addition, conflicting studies show that small meals more often could lead to weight gain. There is surprisingly a lack of studies available on this topic to be able to absolutely say small meals more frequently can control appetite and weight gain.

Chapter 9:
Intermittent Fasting Q&A

Question: What are the restrictions on who should fast?

Answer: There are several medical reasons a person should not fast. For example, people already underweight, are under 18 or are pregnant or nursing. In addition, those with illnesses like diabetes, gout, increased levels of uric acid or are taking medications prescribed by a physician should work with their doctor to make sure fasting is right for them.

Question: Does fasting have side effects?

Answer: Yes, there are several possible side effects. Some are minor inconveniences while others may be more annoying. One of the more serious side effects occurs in extended fasts and with people who have a stressed metabolism. This stress can be caused by surgery or an illness. It is called the "refeeding syndrome" and is very uncommon. 4 days after eating again you may experience pulmonary, cardiac, and neurological disorders if you are suffering from this syndrome.

On the other hand, it is common to experience:

- Heartburn

- Muscle cramps

- Stomach rumblings

- Headaches

- Constipation

Question: What does it take to break a fast?

Answer: It is important to be gentle with yourself when coming out of a fast. The longer you fast, the gentler you need to be. To avoid hurting your stomach, do not gorge yourself on a "victory meal" when your fasting is done. When you first begin fasting it is normal to want to do this but after the first few times of the discomfort, you will learn it is important to resume normal eating.

Question: Are women allowed to fast?

Answer: YES! The problems women face during a fast are similar to the problems men face. The results can also be similar to the results of men; however, some studies have shown that women are more responsive to intermittent fasting than men, making them actually better candidates for this lifestyle! The only exceptions include women that are nursing, pregnant or are underweight.

Question: What is the difference between various intermittent fasts?

Answer: There are many versions of intermittent fasting. Short fasts, which last less than 24 hours, are less effective and more frequent than longer versions. For example, someone who eats for 8 hours and fasts for 16 could do it every day while someone who fasts for 24 hours could do it 2 or 3 times a week.

Question: Do you have to choose one style of intermittent fasting or can you change it throughout the week?

Answer: The body learns to adapt to new patterns so changing up routines can keep it "guessing." But on the flip side, not having a routine can lead to not having a fast at all. So, this all depends on you. If you thrive on routine and stability, then pick one thing and stick to it. If you do well-changing things up and being flexible, then, by all means, keep the body guessing.

Question: What is the best process for starting a fast?

Answer: Some people like to jump into fasting with two feet while others ease in gently, starting off slow and ramping up over time. It all depends on who you are and what makes sense for you. If you are nervous about starting something too drastic, try cutting out a meal or two a couple of times a week and then slowly increasing the time between meals or more days per week. If you don't think you will make a change if you do not fully commit, then plan to go big and stick it out for a pre-determined length of time. It is completely up to you; both starting points work.

Question: Other than water, what options are there for hydration?

Answer: Bone broth is one of the best options for hydration, other than water. This is because it is both filling and nutritious. Consider it as a liquid supplement of important vitamins and minerals. This form of hydration also does well with added sodium to help keep you hydrated. Other beverages that you can consume, like coffee and tea, can help satiate your appetite temporarily but are not as good hydration or full of nutrients.

Question: Is there a relationship between fasting and kidney stones?

Answer: Some people are more predisposed to getting kidney stones. Some situations can create stones. There is no direct correlation between fasting and developing kidney stones; however, it is important to drink plenty of fluids. Ingesting enough salt and water is important to preventing kidney stones.

Question: How can side effects like a bloated stomach or constipation be treated on a fasting day?

Answer: Adding a fiber supplement is a common method for relieving stomach tension and constipation. If this does not work, other laxatives can be taken. Consider taking senna tea or milk of magnesia. This side effect is usual but irritating. Treating this with a softener can help the longevity of the fast and the overall experience.

Question: Is exercise safe during a fast?

Answer: Basically, yes. All daily activities are fine to do while fasting. This includes exercising as well. Body fat is being used to fuel the body during a fast so when you increase your exertion you burn even more fat. But it is important to remember that your body may be feeling tired of this change and the detox that it is going through. Do not overstress your body or your willpower. On non-fast days consider doing more aerobic and intense workouts while on fasting days, choose something gentler like light weight lifting or yoga.

Question: Is reducing calories the same or a form of fasting?

Answer: No. The two concepts are very different from one another. Reducing calories at mealtime or throughout the day are focused on what you are eating; fasting is focused on when you are eating. While fasting does result in a reduction of calories, it is not the primary goal of this method, and there are far more benefits to choosing this lifestyle than just restricting caloric intake.

Question: How much weight can be expected to be lost?

Answer: This varies person to person and intermittent fast to intermittent fast. It is practically guaranteed you will lose weight; however, if you choose to do a shorter fast for less than 24-hours, the weight loss will not be as dramatic than if you had done a 24 or 36 hour fast a couple times a week. In addition, controlling your eating during non-fasting days is important to your weight loss goals as well. Not gorging yourself when you do eat can make sure your body continues to use body fat for energy rather than carbohydrates. This is a historical method for health and weight control that is still relevant today.

Question: Can overweight children or teenagers use intermittent fasting to achieve their weight loss goals?

Answer: No, this is not recommended. Children should never fast. Even teenagers should not fast because their constantly growing bodies need a steady source of nutrients for proper development. Teenagers can do short fasts, for less than 24 hours, but it should be under direct supervision with a doctor. Children who need to lower their weight should do so by reducing daily meals or cutting out unhealthy foods and snacks.

Question: What is the best length of a fast?

Answer: There is no set time limit for a fasting state; however, if you plan to go over 1 week not eating you should partner with a doctor for constant supervision. Some fasting states have gone on for several months, but they did so under medical care. Staying with a fasting time of less than 1 week is best for those that do not or cannot meet often with their doctor. The peak in fasting benefits typically occurs during the third and fourth days so it is possible to get a lot of the benefits without extending further than a week.

Question: When training for a competition or marathon, does fasting or non-fasting days need to correspond with training schedules and is it necessary to take a supplement to help retain muscles?

Answer: Your muscles do not break down while on an intermittent fast. In fact, the research has shown that those that practice intermittent fasting retain more lean muscle than those that lose weight through other dieting methods. This means taking a supplement for muscle growth and recovery is not necessary. As for training, there is a current fitness trend called "fasted state training." This is because the body does not need food to energize itself and when it is burning what you already have rather than what you just put in, you lose more weight and become more in tune with your body. Growth hormones are increased during a fasting state meaning that your muscles will actually grow and recover quicker. Many intermittent fasting regimens used for those doing some form of training are 24-hour fasts. The fast occurs the day before a training day.

Conclusion

Thank for making it through to the end of *Intermittent Fasting: A safe guide to long-lasting weight loss*, let's hope it was informative and able to provide you with all of the tools you need to achieve your goals whatever they may be.

The next step is to begin your journey into this new lifestyle by deciding which method of intermittent fasting is right for you. Maybe you decide to start with a short trial run or maybe you dive right into a "warrior" diet. Whatever method you decide to go with, remember that this is a mental game as much as it is physical. Take time to celebrate your successes. This means that each time you complete a fasting period counts it as a win! You are making a commitment to a healthier and long-lasting way to control your weight, but you will experience many more benefits than that.

Hopefully, you have found the answers to the questions you had regarding intermittent fasting throughout this book. The last chapter was dedicated to just that, after all! There have been several studies on this topic and many more are in the works. This is not a new way of eating and it is not going to go away. Keep on the lookout for new studies and research being released and you will keep up with not only your weight but your health and wellness as well. Stay focused on improving yourself and enjoy your new, healthier life!

Finally, if you found this book useful in any way, a review on Amazon is always appreciated!